The Definitive Keto Vegan Recipe Book

Affordable and tasty keto vegan recipes

Nancy Graham

Please consult a licensed professional before attempting any techniques outlined in this book.

By reading this document, the reader agrees that under no circumstances is the author responsible for any losses, direct or indirect, which are incurred as a result of the use of information contained within this document, including, but not limited to, — errors, omissions, or inaccuracies.

TABLE OF CONTENTS

Low-carb coconut hamburger buns

Preparation Time: 10 minutes - Cooking Time: 20 minutes - Servings: 4

Ingredients:

- 1/2 cup coconut flour - 1 1/2 cups mozzarella cheese, shredded
- 2 tablespoons cream cheese, softened - 2 tablespoons flax meal
- 2 eggs, large - 1 tablespoon baking powder
- 1 tablespoon sesame seeds - 1/2 teaspoon salt

Directions:

1. Preheat your oven to 380°F.
2. Using a mixing bowl, whisk your flax meal, coconut flour, salt and baking soda.
3. In another bowl, put your cream cheese and mozzarella cheese. Microwave your cheese for 45 seconds to a minute. Stir it and microwave once more until it becomes melted.
4. Beat your eggs, adding into the first bowl which has the dry ingredients. Add the cheese too to the bowl. You can use your hand mixer to make the dough.

5. Separate the dough into four equal portions. Use these portions to make the buns and sprinkle sesame seeds. Press the seeds to prevent them from falling out.

6. Line the baking sheet with parchment paper and place your buns.

7. Bake for 20 minutes or until they brown on the outside.

8. Leave them to cool.

Nutrition: Calories 218 / Carbohydrates 7.2 g / Fats 13.5 g / Protein 17 g

Low-carb dinner rolls

Preparation Time: 10 minutes - Cooking Time: 10 minutes - Servings: 6

Ingredients:

- 1 cup almond flour - 1/4 cup flaxseed, ground
- 1 cup Mozzarella, shredded - 1 oz. cream cheese
- 1/2 teaspoon baking soda - 1 egg

Directions:

1. Preheat your oven to 400°F.
2. Using a microwave-safe mixing bowl, microwave cream cheese and the mozzarella for a minute. Stir them till they become smooth.
3. Add eggs in the bowl while stirring to mix well.
4. In another clean bowl, put your almond flour, baking soda and flaxseed and mix the dry ingredients.
5. Pour your egg and cheese mix into the bowl with dry ingredients. Use your hand mixer or hands to make dough by kneading.
6. Slightly wet your hands with coconut oil or olive oil and roll your dough to six balls.
7. Top them with sesame seeds and place them on the parchment paper.

8. Bake them for 10 minutes. A golden brown look will indicate that they are done.

9. Leave them to cool.

Nutrition: Calories 219 / Carbohydrates 5.6 g / Fats 18 g / Protein 10.7 g

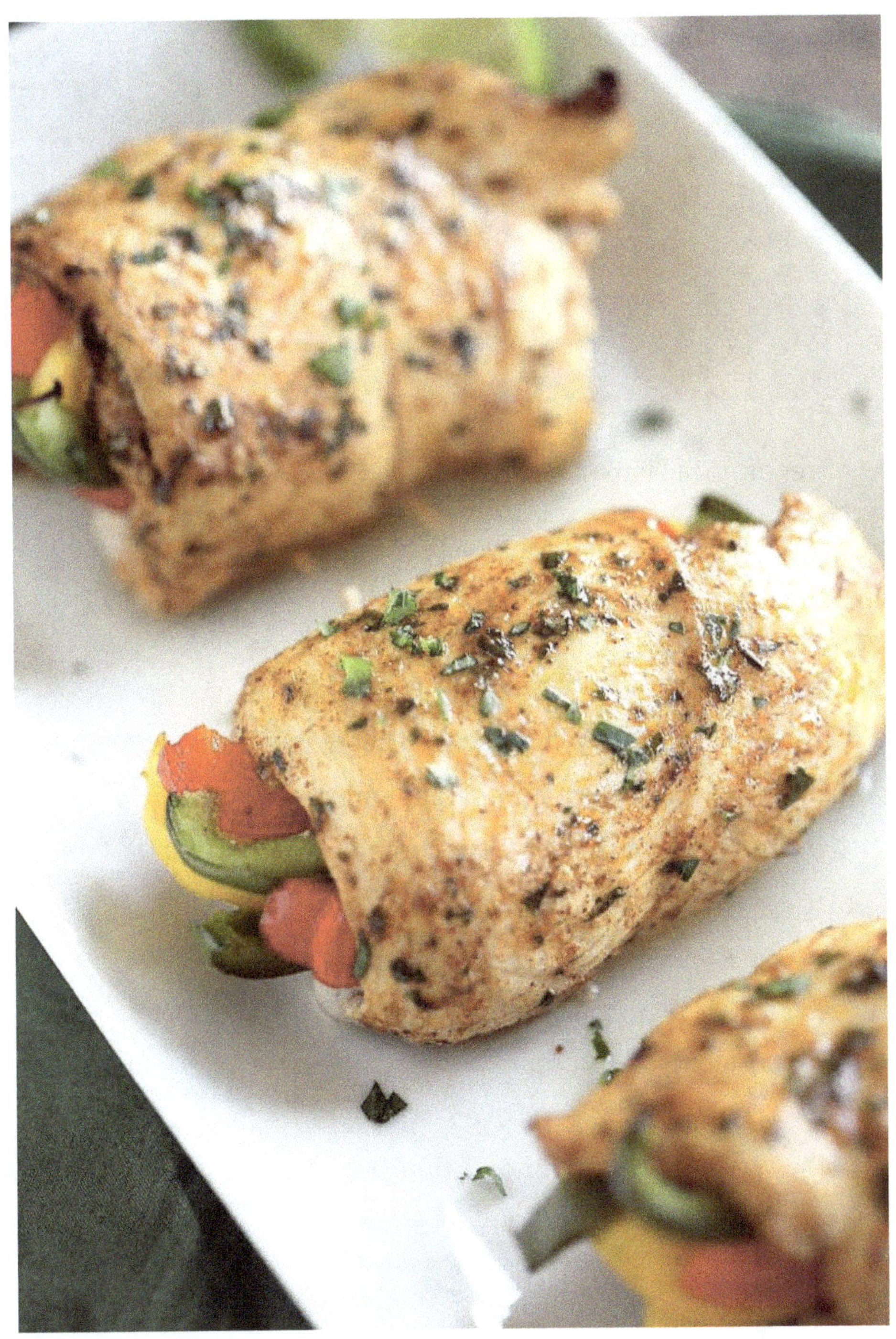

Low-carb clover rolls

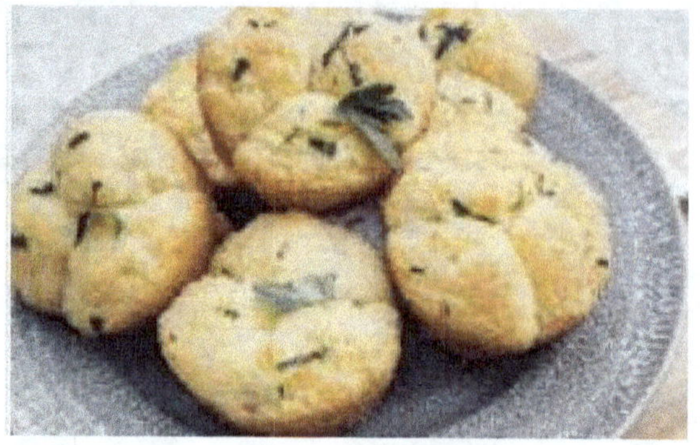

Preparation Time: 10 minutes - Cooking Time: 20 minutes - Servings: 8

Ingredients:

- I/3 cup coconut flour
- 1 1/2 cup mozzarella cheese, shredded
- 1 1/2 teaspoon baking powder
- 1/4 cup parmesan cheese, grated
- 2 ounces cream cheese
- 2 eggs, large

Directions:

1. Preheat your oven to 350°F.
2. Put your almond flour and baking powder in a clean bowl and mix.

3. Using another bowl, put your Mozzarella and cream cheese and microwave for a minute. Stir it well after it melts.
4. Add eggs to the cheese and stir.
5. Add the egg-cheese mix to the bowl with dry ingredients and mix thoroughly.
6. Wet your hands and knead dough into a sticky ball.
7. Put the dough ball on the parchment paper and slice into fourths.
8. Slice each fourth or quarter into 6 smaller portions.
9. Roll each small portion into balls.
10. Roll the balls into the parmesan cheese light for them to coat it.
11. Grease your muffin pan and place 3 dough balls in each cup of the pan.
12. Bake it for 20 minutes at 350°F.

Nutrition: Calories 283 / Carbohydrates 6 g / Fats 21 g / Protein 16 g

Keto bread rolls

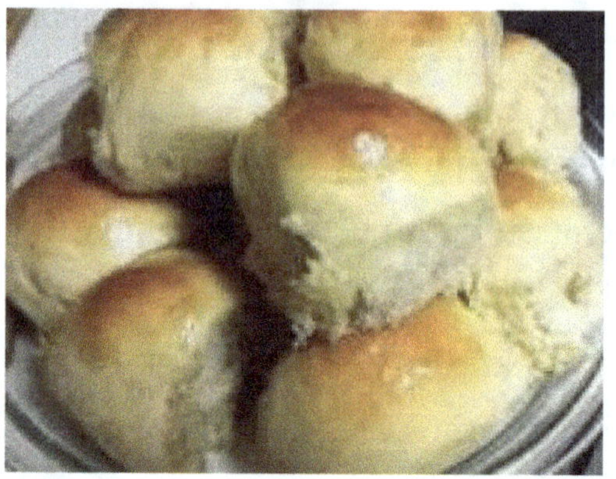

Preparation Time: 10 minutes - Cooking Time: 20 minutes - Servings: 8

Ingredients:

- 1 1/3 cups almond flour
- 1 1/2 cups shredded mozzarella cheese, part skim
- 2 oz. cream cheese, full fat
- 1 1/2 tablespoon baking powder, aluminum free
- 2 tablespoons coconut flour
- 3 eggs

Directions:

1. Preheat your oven to 350°F
2. In a clean bowl, put almond flour, coconut flour and baking powder. Mix well and set it aside.

3. Using a microwave-safe bowl, put the cream cheese and mozzarella in it and microwave for 30 seconds. Remove the bowl, stir and microwave again for 30 seconds. This should go on until the cheese has entirely melted.
4. Using a food processor add the cheese, the eggs and flour mix. Process at high speed for uniformity of the dough. (It is normally sticky.)
5. Knead the dough into a dough ball and separate it into 8 equal pieces. Slightly wet your hands with oil for this step.
6. Roll each piece with your palms to form a ball and place each ball on the baking sheet. (should be 2 inches apart)
7. In a bowl, add the remaining egg and whisk. Brush the egg wash on the rolls.
8. Bake for 20 minutes or until they are golden brown.

Nutrition: Calories 216 / Carbohydrates 6 g / Fats 16 g / Protein 11 g

Seeded Buns

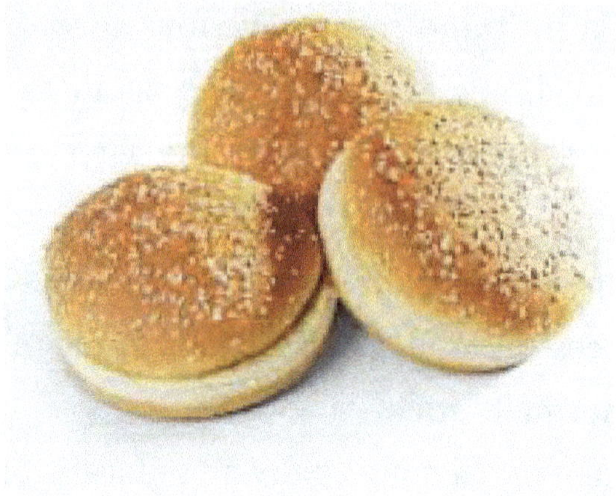

Preparation Time: 10 minutes - Cooking Time: 35 minutes - Servings: 6

Ingredients:

- 1 cup almond flour
- 2 tsp. baking powder
- 3 egg whites
- 1.25 cup hot water
- 2 tbsp. sesame seeds
- 5 tbsp. psyllium husk powder
- 1 tsp. salt
- 2 tsp. apple cider vinegar
- medium saucepan
- standard sized flat sheet

Directions:

1. Warm the water in a saucepan until it starts to bubble. Transfer to a glass dish.
2. In the meantime, prepare a flat sheet with a layer of baking lining and set to the side.
3. Blend the water with the almond flour, baking powder, psyllium husk, salt, and apple cider vinegar until it becomes a thick consistency.
4. Section into 6 equal portions and form mounds.
5. Apply pressure to flatten the mounds to approximately 1 inch thick.
6. Arrange on the prepped flat sheet and glaze with the melted butter.
7. Dust with the sesame seeds and heat for approximately 35 minutes.
8. Serve immediately and enjoy!

Nutrition: Calories 73 / Carbohydrates 7 g / Fats 3 g / Protein 3 g

Moutabelle with Keto Flatbread

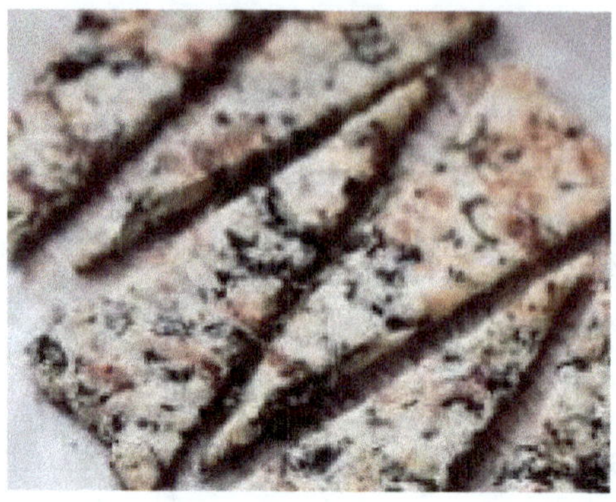

Preparation Time: 20 minutes - Cooking Time: 20 minutes - Servings: 6

Ingredients:

For the Moutabelle

- 500 grams Eggplant - 75 grams White Onion
- 10 grams Flat Parsley - 2 tbsp. tahini paste
- 2 tbsp. Lemon Juice - ¼ cup Olive Oil
- Salt, to taste - Pepper, to taste

For the Flatbread:

- ½ cup Almond Flour - 2 tbsp. Psyllium Husk
- ¼ tsp Baking Soda - pinch of Salt
- 1 tbsp. Olive Oil - 1 cup Lukewarm Water

Directions:

Prepare the Flatbread:

1. Whisk together the almond flour, psyllium husk, baking soda, and salt in a bowl.
2. Add in the water and olive oil.
3. Knead until everything comes together into a smooth dough.
4. Leave to rest for about 15 minutes.
5. Divide the dough into 6 equal-sized portions.
6. Roll each portion into a ball, then flatten with a rolling pin in between sheets of parchment paper.
7. Refrigerate until ready to use.
8. To cook, heat in a non-stick pan for 2-3 minutes per side.

Prepare the moutabelle:

9. Split each eggplant in half lengthwise. Brush with olive oil and season with salt.
10. Grill over high heat until fully cooked. Set aside until cool enough to handle.
11. Peel the grilled eggplants, and transfer the flesh to a blender or food processor. Add in remaining ingredients and process until

smooth. You may add a little warm water if it is too thick to process.

Nutrition: Calories 171 / Carbohydrates 9 g / Fats 15 g / Protein 2 g

Vegetable Latkes Spiked with Curry

Preparation Time: 15 minutes - Cooking Time: 6 minutes - Servings: 6

Ingredients:

- 100 grams Carrots, spiralized
- 100 grams Zucchini, spiralized
- 100 grams Cauliflower, minced
- 50 grams minced White Onion
- 5 grams Parsley, chopped
- ¼ cup Almond Flour
- 1 tbsp. Flax Seeds, soaked in 2 tbsp. Water
- 2 tsp Curry Powder
- ½ tsp Salt
- 2 tbsp. Olive Oil plus more for frying

Directions:

1. In a bowl, mix almond flour, egg, parsley, onions, curry powder, and salt.
2. In a non-stick skillet over medium heat, heat olive oil.
3. Using a spoon, add vegetable mixture to the hot oil, while you shape every latke like an egg ring.
4. Over medium heat, fry each side for about 3 minutes.

5. Use paper towels to drain.

Nutrition: Calories 123 / Carbohydrates 5 g / Fats 12 g / Protein 2 g

Vegan Cheese Fondue

Preparation Time: 5 minutes - Cooking Time: 20 minutes - Servings: 4

Ingredients:

- 70 grams Raw Cashews - 1 tbsp. Nutritional Yeast
- 1 tsp Garlic Powder - 2 tsp Cider Vinegar
- 2 tbsp. Gelatin - 1 tbsp. Turmeric Powder
- 1 tsp Salt - cups Water - 200 grams Zucchini, cut into sticks

Directions:

1. Boil cashews over high heat in a saucepan for 14 minutes.
2. Blend garlic powder, cashews, gelatin, vinegar, turmeric powder, water, yeast, and salt until smooth.
3. Add the puree to a saucepot and boil for about 4-5 minutes, while constantly stirring. Stir until the mixture is smooth.
4. Put it to a fondue pot and enjoy alongside zucchini sticks.

Nutrition: Calories 126 / Carbohydrates 9 g / Fats 8 g / Protein 6 g

Chocolate Peanut Butter Cookies

Preparation Time: 20 minutes - Cooking Time: 10 minutes - Servings: 14

Ingredients:

- ½ cup Peanut Butter, melted
- 3 tbsp. Coconut Oil
- ½ cup Vegan Semi-Sweet Chocolate Chips
- ½ cup Erythritol
- ½ cup Coconut Milk
- 1 tsp Vanilla Extract
- 2 cups Almond Flour
- ½ teaspoon Salt
- ½ teaspoon Baking Soda

Directions:

1. Stir together peanut butter, coconut oil, vanilla extract erythritol, and coconut milk in a bowl.
2. In a separate bowl, whisk together baking soda, flour, and salt.
3. Stir the dry mixture into the wet mixture.
4. Fold the chocolate chips in.
5. Shape dough into cookies and arrange on a baking tray lined with parchment paper.

6. Bake for 10 minutes at 375°F.

Nutrition: Calories 179 / Carbohydrates 5 g / Fats 16 g / Protein 5 g

Sweet Potato Toast

Preparation Time: 3 minutes - Cooking Time: 20 minutes - Servings: 4

Ingredients:

- 1 Ripe avocado
- 1 Large sweet potato
- Pepper and salt
- ½ cup Roughly-chopped pistachios
- 3 tbsp. Olive oil
- Crushed red pepper flakes

Directions:

1. Warm up the oven to 400°F. Prepare a baking sheet with aluminum foil.
2. Slice the potato into 1/4-inch rounds. Arrange on the baking sheet and toss it with the oil, salt, and pepper.
3. Bake for 20 minutes and garnish with the avocado and pistachios. Add a few pepper flakes.

Nutrition: Calories 132 / Carbohydrates 7 g / Fats 11 g / Protein 2 g

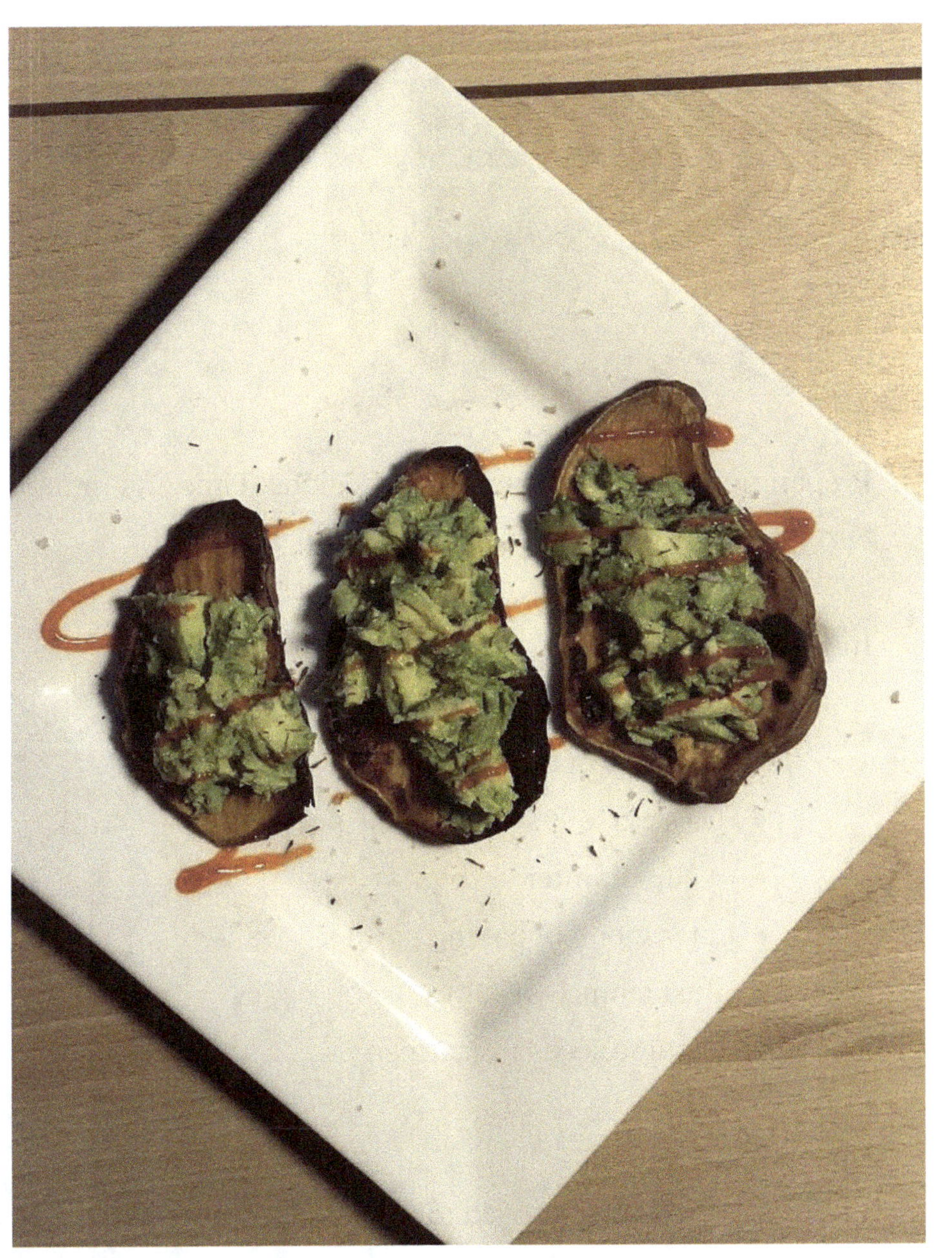

Never Fear Thin Bagels Pieces

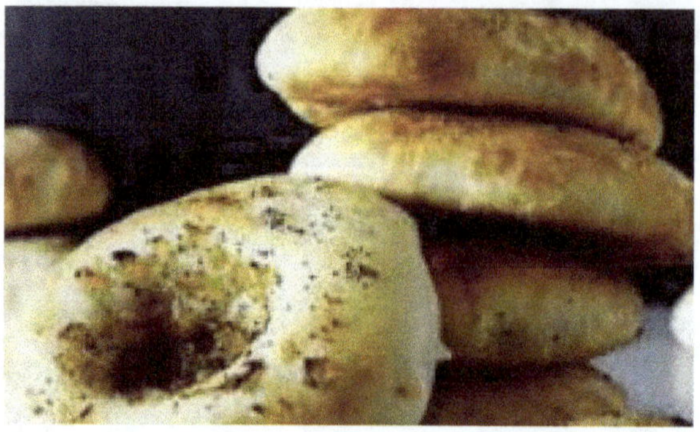

Preparation Time: 10 minutes - Cooking Time: 40 minutes - Servings: 8

Ingredients

- 3 tablespoon of ground flaxseed
- ½ a cup of tahini
- ½ a cup of Psyllium Husk powder
- 1 cup of water
- 1 teaspoon of baking powder
- Just a pinch of salt
- Sesame seeds for garnish

Directions

1. Preheat your oven to 375 degrees Fahrenheit
2. Take a mixing bowl and add Psyllium Husk, baking powder, ground flax seeds, salt and keep whisking until combined

3. Add water to the dry mix and keep mixing until the water has been absorbed fully
4. Add tahini and keep mixing until the dough forms
5. Knead well
6. Form patties from the dough that have a diameter of 4 inches and a thickness of ¼ inch
7. Lay them carefully on your baking tray
8. Cut up a small hole in the middle
9. Add sesame seeds on top
10. Bake for 40 minutes until a golden brown texture is seen
11. Cut them in half and toast if you like
12. Top them up with your favorite Keto-Vegan compliant spread
13. Enjoy!

Nutrition: Calories: 129 / Fat: 10g / Carbs: 2g / Protein: 4g

Veggie Wraps with Glorious Tahini Sauce

Preparation Time: 10 minutes - Cooking Time: 0 minutes - Servings: 8

Ingredients

- ¼ cup of sliced carrots
- 2 tablespoon of sauerkraut
- 2 tablespoon of tahini sauce

Directions

1. De-vein your leaves and wash them well
2. Add carrots, sauerkraut and wrap them up well
3. Pour the sauce directly/use as a dip
4. Enjoy!

Nutrition: Calories: 120 / Fat: 8g / Carbs: 6g / Protein: 4g

Very White Chocolate Peanut Butter Bites

Preparation Time: 110 minutes - Cooking Time: 0 minutes - Servings: 8

Ingredients

- ½ a cup of cacao butter
- ½ a cup of salted peanut butter
- 3 tablespoon of Stevia
- 4 tablespoon of powdered coconut milk
- 2 teaspoon of vanilla extract

Directions

1. Set your double boiler on low heat
2. Melt the cacao butter and peanut butter together and stir in vanilla extract
3. Take another bowl and add powdered coconut powder and Stevia
4. Stir one tablespoon at a time of the mixture into the vanilla extract mixture
5. Portion the mixture into silicone molds or lined up muffin tins and chill them for 90 minutes
6. Remove and enjoy it!

Nutrition: Calories: 77 / Fat: 7g / Carbs: 8g / Protein: 2g

Coconut Blueberries Ice Cream

Preparation Time: 15 min. - Cooking Time: 0 minutes - Servings: 2

Ingredients:

- half cup fresh blueberries
- 4 tbsp. shredded coconut
- 1 cup unsweetened coconut milk
- 5 tbsp. coconut butter
- 15 drops of stevia
- 2 tbsp. vanilla

Directions:

1. Pulse the blueberries, coconut milk, coconut butter, shredded coconut, stevia and vanilla using a blender.
2. Spoon the mixture into the ice cream maker and process for 1 hour or according to manufacturer's instructions.
3. Spoon the blueberries mixture into the silicone molds or an ice tray.
4. Freeze the coconut and blueberries ice cream for overnight and then serve.

Nutrition: Calories: 164 / Total fat: 29 oz. / Total carbohydrates: 9 oz. / Protein: 13 oz.

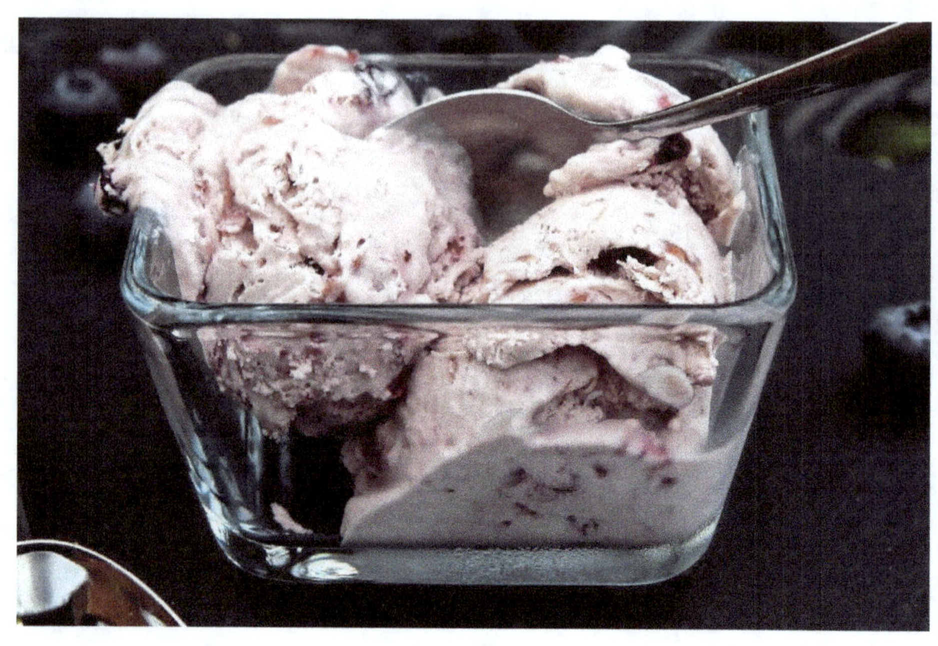

Walnuts Cakes

Preparation Time: 15 min. - Cooking Time: 5 min. - Servings: 2

Ingredients:

- 1 cup walnuts, ground
- 10 oz. unsweetened dark chocolate
- half cup coconut oil
- 7 tbsp. cocoa powder
- 3 tbsp. erythritol
- 5 tbsp. coconut butter
- 1 tbsp. vanilla
- salt

Directions:

1. Melt the coconut oil in the microwave for 5 minutes and combine it with the cocoa powder, vanilla, erythritol and salt.
2. Pour the mixture into the bowl and place in the fridge for around 10 minutes.
3. Spoon half teaspoon of coconut butter and add the walnuts and then mix well.
4. Spoon the mixture into paper muffin cups.
5. Melt the dark chocolate on medium heat for around 5 min., stirring all the time.
6. Cool the mixture and slowly pour it over the cakes.

7. The cakes should be placed in the fridge for at least 2 hours.

Nutrition: Calories: 162 / Total fat: 22 oz. / Total carbohydrates: 4 oz. / Protein: 10 oz.

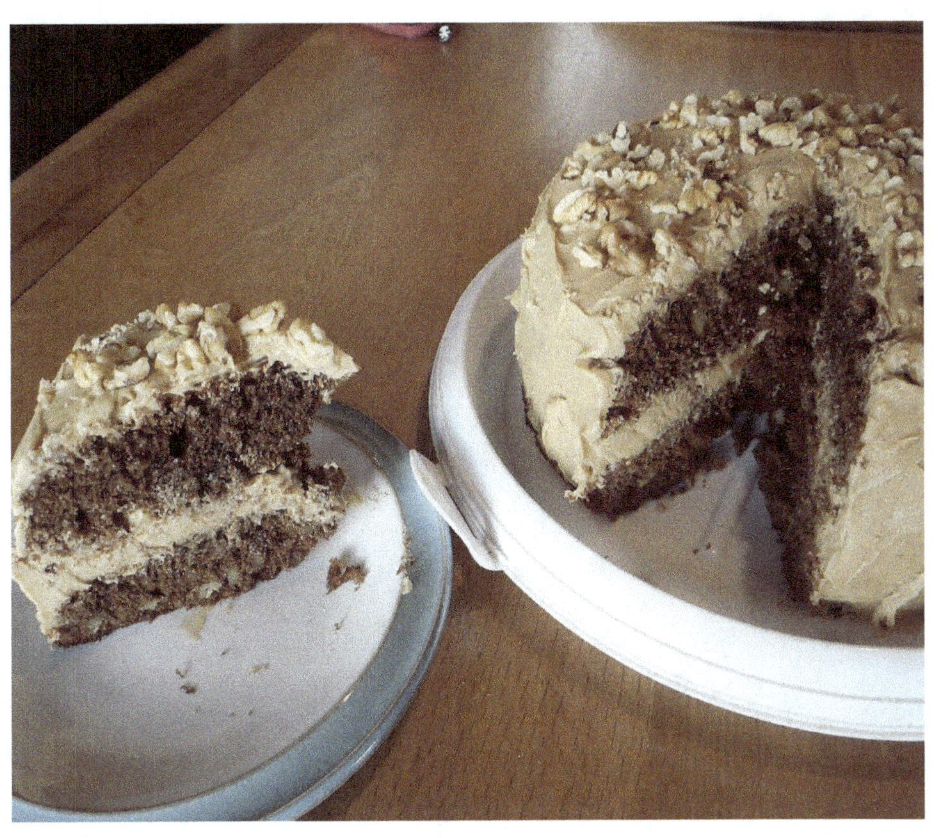

Raspberries Mousse

Preparation Time: 5 min. - Cooking Time: 15 min. - Servings: 4

Ingredients:

- 1 cup fresh raspberries
- half cup almond milk
- 10 oz. coconut butter
- 3 tbsp. erythritol
- 2 tbsp. vanilla

Directions:

1. Boil the almond milk in a pan over low heat for 5 min.
2. Combine the raspberries with the almond milk and pulse well using a blender.
3. Use an electric hand mixer and beat together the raspberries mixture, coconut butter, erythritol and vanilla in a mixing bowl until the homogenous mass.
4. Pour the raspberries mixture into the jars or glasses.
5. Freeze the raspberries mixture for around 20 min. and serve.

Nutrition: Calories: 195 / Total fat: 29 oz. / Total carbohydrates: 3 oz. / Protein: 11 oz.

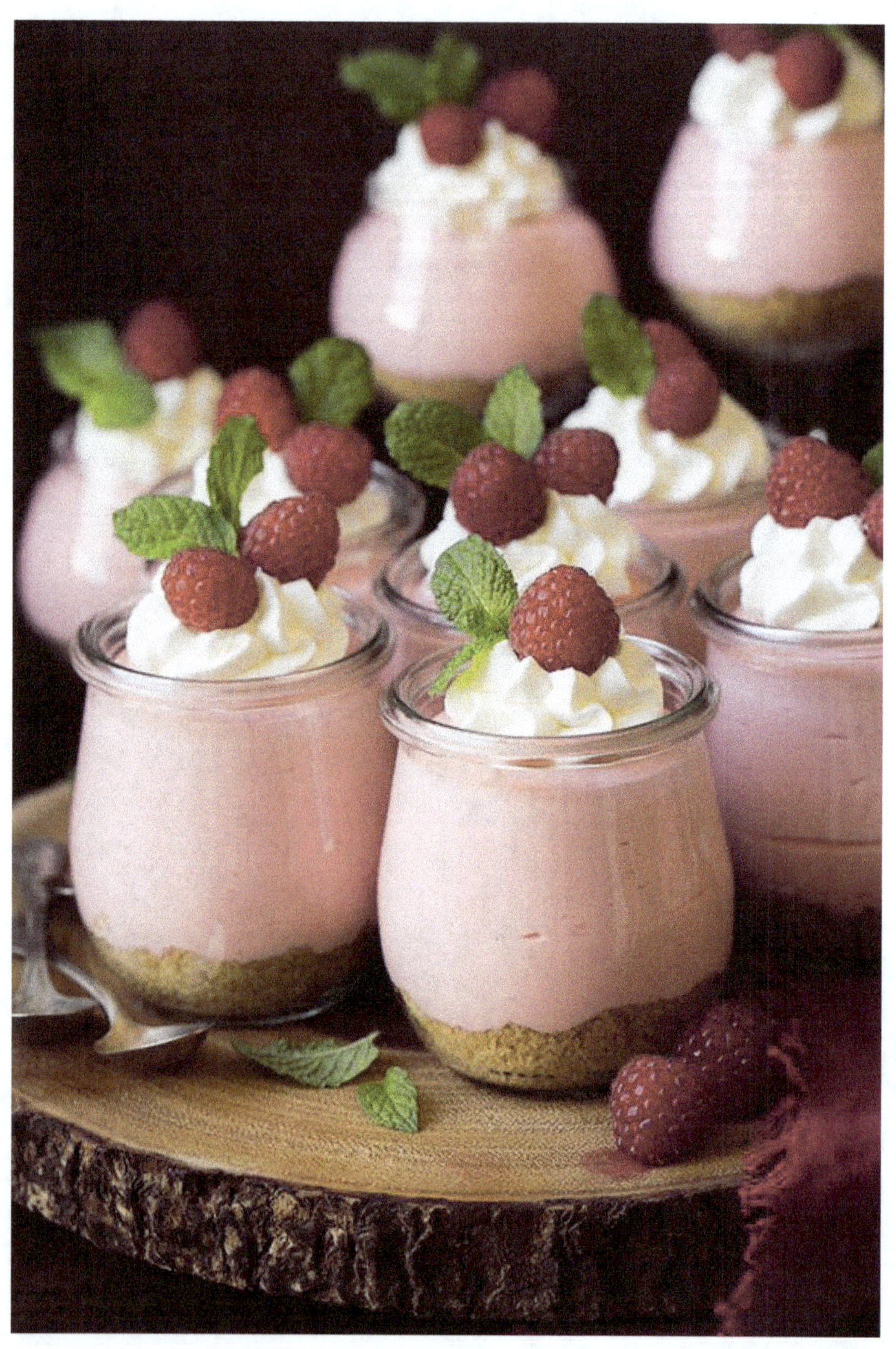

Vegan Orange Muffins

Preparation Time: 15 min. - Cooking Time: 0 minutes - Servings: 2

Ingredients:

- 2 tbsp. pure orange extract
- 2 tsp. orange zest
- 7 tbsp. coconut butter
- 5 oz. coconut oil
- 5 oz. cocoa powder
- 15 drops of stevia

Directions:

1. In a bowl, combine the coconut butter, coconut oil, orange extract, orange zest, cocoa powder and stevia.
2. Place all the ingredients into a food processor and blend until they have a smooth and creamy consistency.
3. Spoon the mixture into paper muffin cups and place in the fridge for around 2 hours and then serve.

Nutrition: Calories: 161 / Total fat: 25 oz. / Total carbohydrates: 7 oz. / Protein: 11 oz.

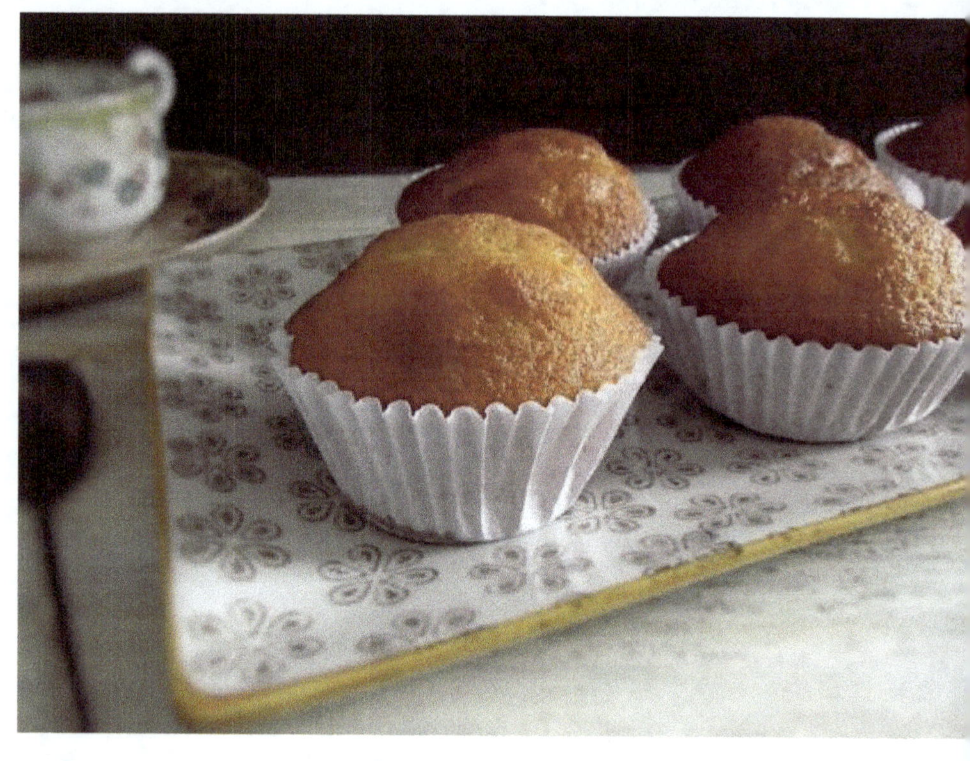

Coconut Keto Vegan Ice Cream

Preparation Time: 5 min. - Cooking Time: 1 h. 20 min. - Servings: 4

Ingredients:

- 15 oz. coconut cream
- 5 oz. cocoa powder
- half cup almond milk
- 4 tbsp. powdered erythritol
- shredded coconut
- vanilla

Directions:

1. Place the coconut cream, cocoa powder, shredded coconut, erythritol and vanilla into a pot and heat gently for 10 minutes, stirring, warming up until dissolved.
2. Use an electric hand mixer and whisk the almond milk and slowly pour the sweet coconut cream mixture, stirring all the time.
3. Pour the almond-coconut mixture into the pot and heat gently for 10 minutes, stirring, warming up and then cool.

4. Spoon the mixture into the ice cream maker and process for 1 hour or according to manufacturer's instructions and freeze for at least 3 hours.

Nutrition: Calories: 159 / Total fat: 29 oz. / Total carbohydrates: 6 oz. / Protein: 13 oz.

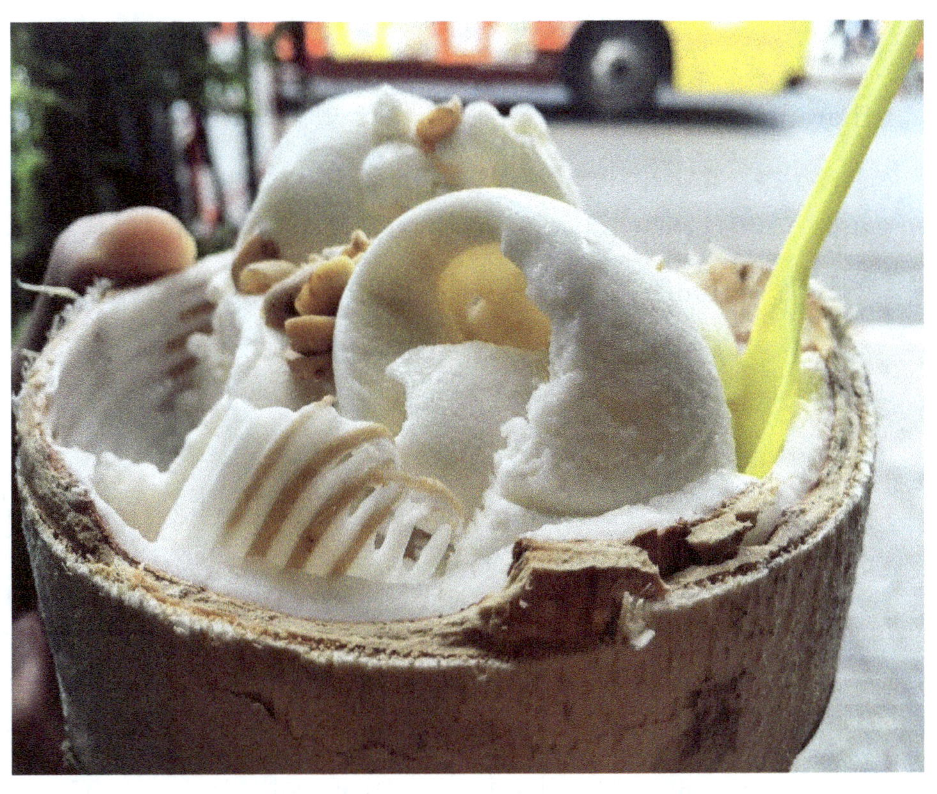

Lemon Bars

Preparation Time: 10 min. - Cooking Time: 1 h. 5 min. - Servings: 5

Ingredients:

- 4 tbsp. lemon zest, minced - 8 oz. coconut butter
- 4 tbsp. coconut cream - 1 cup almond flour
- half cup silken tofu - 4 tbsp. powdered erythritol
- 4 tsp. baking soda - vanilla

Directions:

1. Melt the coconut butter on medium heat for around 5 minutes, stirring all the time.
2. Combine the coconut butter, half cup of the almond flour, silken tofu, 2 tsp. baking soda, vanilla and 2 tbsp. of the powdered erythritol in a mixing bowl, mashing with a fork until smooth.
3. Spoon the mixture into the baking tray and bake for 30 minutes at 310 degree - 320 degree Fahrenheit.
4. Now let's start the filling by combining the lemon zest, coconut cream, remaining erythritol, baking soda and almond flour.
5. Beat together the filling mixture, in a mixing bowl, using an electric hand mixer.

6. Then, pour the lemon filling mixture onto the cooled almond crust and bake for 30 minutes at 320 degree-330 degree Fahrenheit.
7. Then cool, cut into pieces and serve with the lemon slices on top and orange juice.

Nutrition: Calories: 159 / Total fat: 49 oz. / Total carbohydrates: 9 oz. / Protein: 15 oz.

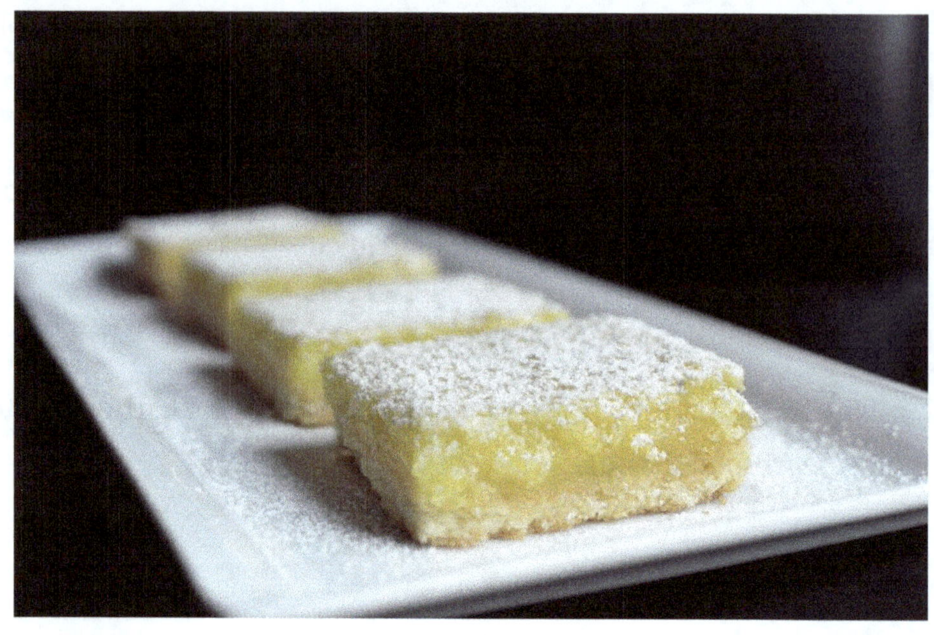

Coconut Pineapple Ice Cream

Preparation Time: 15 min. - Cooking Time: 0 minutes - Servings: 4

Ingredients:

- 3 tsp. pure pineapple extract - 1 can pineapples
- 1 cup unsweetened coconut milk - 5 tbsp. coconut butter
- 3 tbsp. erythritol - 2 tbsp. vanilla

Directions:

1. Pulse the pineapple extract, coconut milk, coconut butter, erythritol and vanilla using a blender.
2. Cut the canned pineapples into cubes and combine with the pineapple mixture.
3. Spoon the mixture into the ice cream maker and process for 1 hour or according to manufacturer's instructions.
4. Spoon the pineapples mixture into the silicone molds or an ice tray.
5. Freeze the pineapples ice cream for overnight and then serve.

Nutrition: Calories: 154 / Total fat: 34 oz. / Total carbohydrates: 8 oz. / Protein: 14 oz.

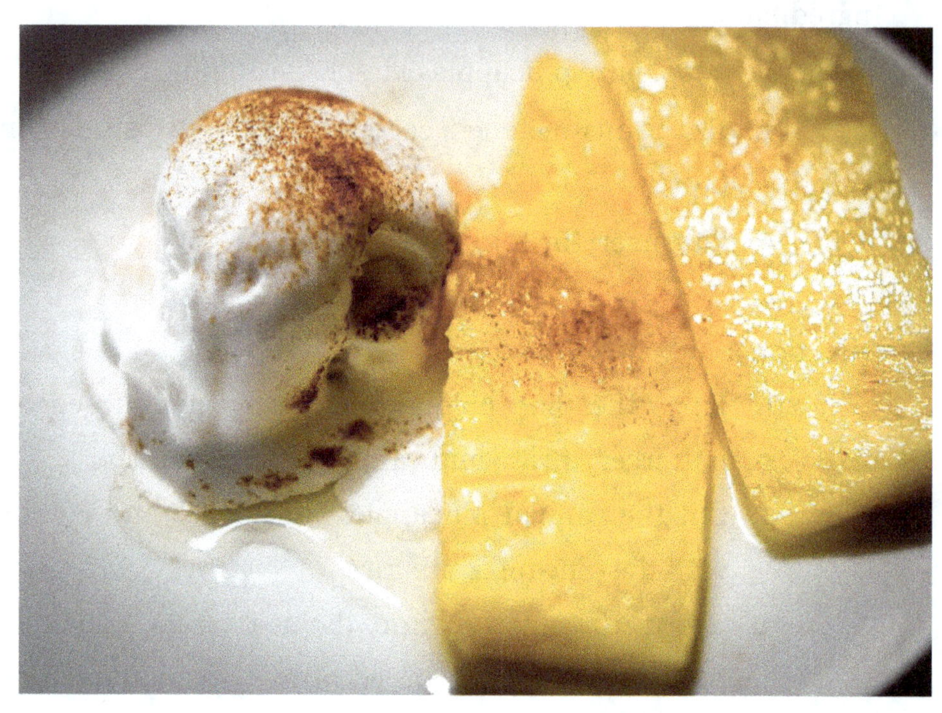

Almond Butter, Oat and Protein Energy Balls

Preparation Time: 1 hour and 10 minutes - Cooking Time: 3 minutes - Servings: 4

Ingredients:

- 1 cup rolled oats
- ½ cup honey
- 2 ½ scoops of vanilla protein powder
- 1 cup almond butter
- Chia seeds for rolling

Directions:

1. Take a skillet pan, place it over medium heat, add butter and honey, stir and cook for 2 minutes until warm.
2. Transfer the mixture into a bowl, stir in protein powder until mixed, and then stir in oatmeal until combined.
3. Shape the mixture into balls, roll them into chia seeds, then arrange them on a cookie sheet and refrigerate for 1 hour until firm.
4. Serve straight away

Nutrition: Calories: 200 Cal / Fat: 10 g / Carbs: 21 g / Protein: 7 g / Fiber: 4 g

Mango Ice Cream

Preparation Time: 5 minutes - Cooking Time: 0 minutes - Servings: 1

Ingredients:

- 2 frouncesen bananas, sliced
- 1 cup diced frouncesen mango

Directions:

1. Place all the ingredients in a food processor and pulse for 2 minutes until smooth.
2. Distribute the ice cream mixture between two bowls and then serve immediately.

Nutrition: Calories: 74 Cal / Fat: 0 g / Carbs: 17 g / Protein: 0 g / Fiber: 4 g

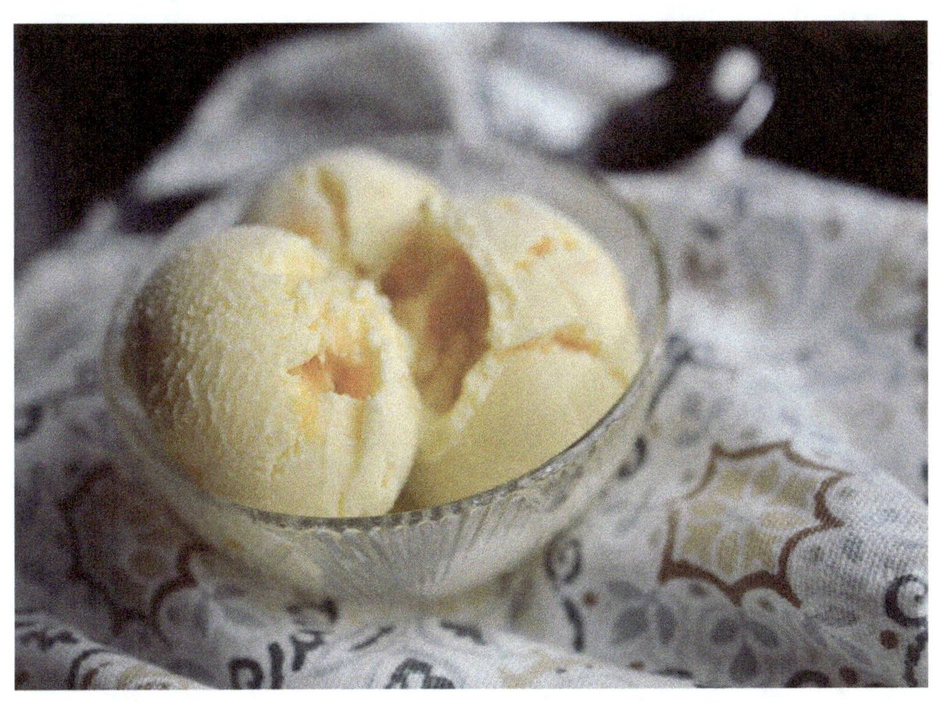

Chocolate and Avocado Truffles

Preparation Time: 1 hour and 10 minutes - Cooking Time: 1 minute - Servings: 18

Ingredients:

- 1 medium avocado, ripe
- 2 tablespoons cocoa powder
- 10 ounces of dark chocolate chips

Directions:

1. Scoop out the flesh from avocado, place it in a bowl, then mash with a fork until smooth, and stir in 1/2 cup chocolate chips.
2. Place remaining chocolate chips in a heatproof bowl and microwave for 1 minute until chocolate has melted, stirring halfway.
3. Add melted chocolate into avocado mixture, stir well until blended, and then refrigerate for 1 hour.
4. Then shape the mixture into balls, 1 tablespoon of mixture per ball, and roll in cocoa powder until covered.
5. Serve straight away.

Nutrition: Calories: 59 Cal / Fat: 4 g / Carbs: 7 g / Protein: 0 g / Fiber: 1 g

Coconut Oil Cookies

Preparation Time: 10 minutes - Cooking Time: 10 minutes - Servings: 15

Ingredients:

- 3 1/4 cup oats - 1/2 teaspoons salt
- 2 cups coconut Sugar
- 1 teaspoons vanilla extract, unsweetened
- 1/4 cup cocoa powder
- 1/2 cup liquid Coconut Oil
- 1/2 cup peanut butter
- 1/2 cup cashew milk

Directions:

1. Take a saucepan, place it over medium heat, add all the ingredients except for oats and vanilla, stir until mixed, and then bring the mixture to boil.
2. Simmer the mixture for 4 minutes, mixing frequently, then remove the pan from heat and stir in vanilla.
3. Add oats, stir until well mixed and then scoop the mixture on a plate lined with wax paper.
4. Serve straight away.

Nutrition: Calories: 112 Cal / Fat: 6.5 g / Carbs: 13 g / Protein: 1.4 g / Fiber: 0.1 g

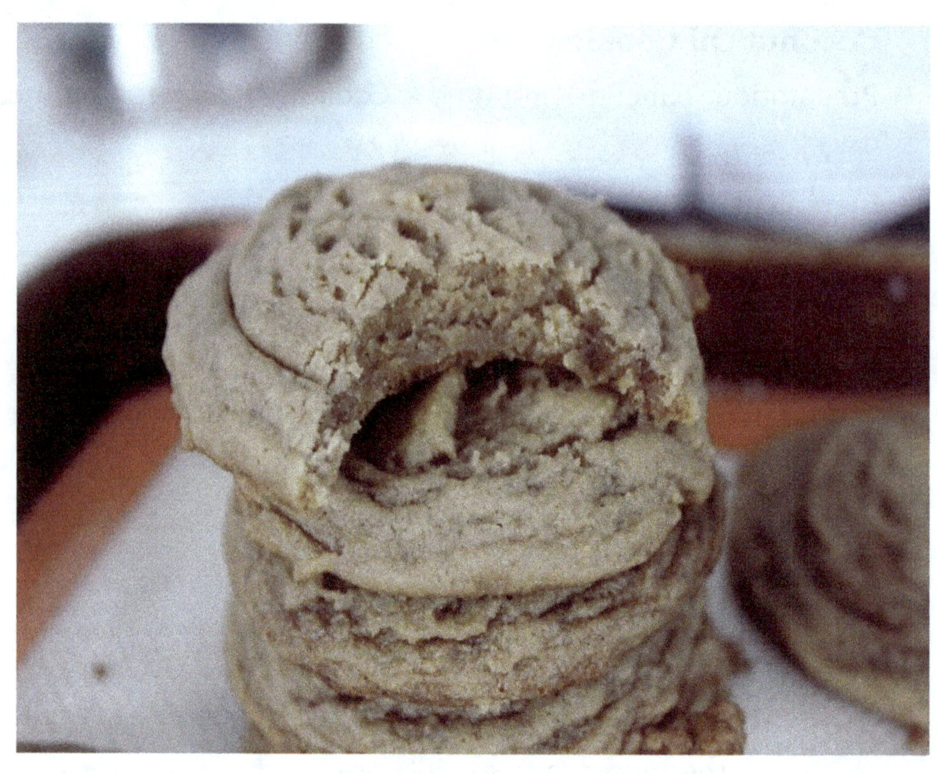

Dark Chocolate Raspberry Ice Cream

Preparation Time: 5 minutes - Cooking Time: 0 minute - Servings: 2

Ingredients:

- 2 frouncesen bananas, sliced
- ¼ cup fresh raspberries
- 2 tablespoons cocoa powder, unsweetened
- 2 tablespoons raspberry jelly

Directions:

1. Place all the ingredients in a food processor, except for berries and pulse for 2 minutes until smooth.
2. Distribute the ice cream mixture between two bowls, stir in berries until combined, and then serve immediately.

Nutrition: Calories: 104 Cal / Fat: 0 g / Carbs: 25 g / Protein: 0 g / Fiber: 5 g

Roasted Almond Nuts

Preparation Time: 5 Minutes - Cooking Time: 10 Minutes - Servings: 6

Ingredients

- One (1) teaspoon of ground cumin
- One (1) teaspoon of salt
- One (1) cup of walnuts
- One (1) teaspoon of paprika powder
- One (1) tablespoon of coconut oil

Directions:

1. Put all the ingredients into a medium sized pan and cook on medium-high heat for 10 minutes, stirring all the while.
2. Set aside to cool for a few minutes before serving as a snack.

Note: You can store the nuts in an airtight container at room temperature.

Nutrition: Calories: 285

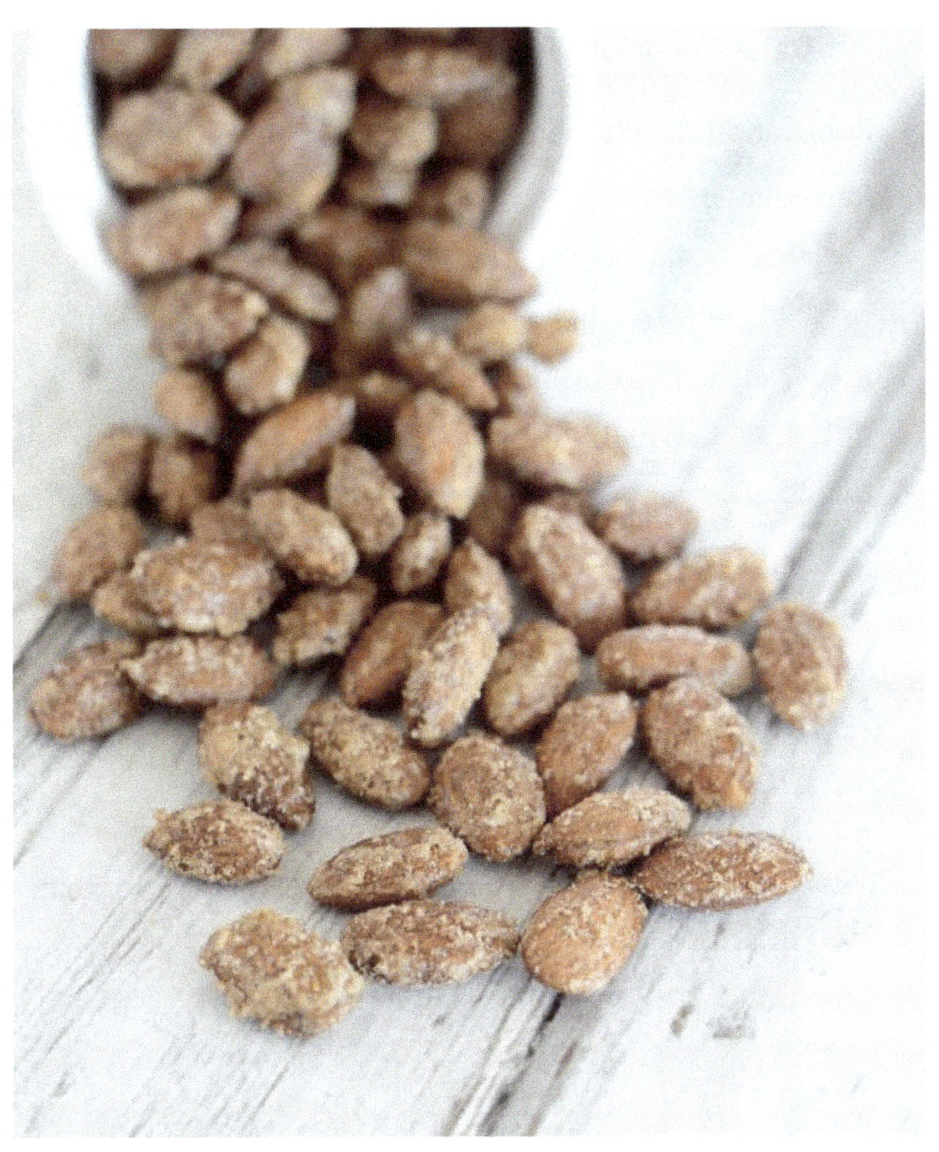

No-Bake Coconut Chia Macaroons

Preparation Time: 2 hours - Cooking Time: - Servings: 6

Ingredients:

- 1 cup Shredded Coconut
- 2 tbsp. Chia Seeds
- ½ cup Coconut Cream
- ½ cup Erythritol

Directions:

1. Combine all ingredients in a bowl. Mix until well combined.
2. Chill the mixture for about half an hour.
3. Once set, scoop the mixture into serving portions and roll into balls.
4. Return to the chiller for another hour.

Nutrition: Kcal per serve: 129 / Fat: 12 g. (80%) / Protein: 2 g. (5%) / Carbs: 5 g. (15%)

Keto Vegan Granola Bars

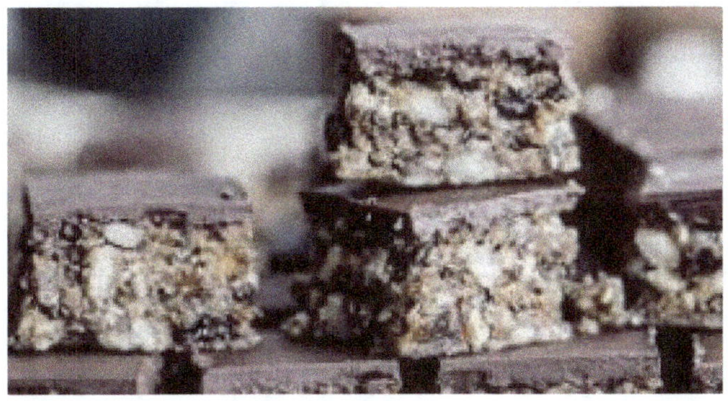

Preparation Time: 10 Minutes - Cooking Time: 60 Minutes - Servings: 6 – Calories : 262

Ingredients

Toppings;

- 25 grab of dark chocolate
- One (1) tablespoon of coconut oil
- Half a teaspoon of peanut butter nut base;
- One (1) teaspoon of collagen
- Two (2) tablespoons of sweetener
- A quarter cup of sliced pecans + half a tablespoon extra
- Four (4) tablespoons of coconut oil
- A quarter cup of pumpkin seeds

- Half a cup of dried strawberries, cranberries and blueberries
- A quarter cup of sliced almonds + one(1) tablespoon extra
- Half a tablespoon of cinnamon
- Four (4) tablespoons of peanut butter
- One (1) tablespoon of chia seeds
- Half a tablespoon of vanilla extract
- A quarter cup of shredded coconut (unsweetened)
- A quarter cup of flaxseed flour
- A quarter cup of sliced walnuts + one (1) tablespoon extra.

Note: All the extras are for decorating the top of the bars, do not add to the main recipe.

Directions:

1. Put the collagen, sweetener, cinnamon, peanut butter, vanilla extract and two tablespoons of coconut oil into a medium sized mixing bowl. Stir until well combined.
2. Put into the microwave for 1-2 minutes, removing once to stir then microwave for another minute, then set aside.
3. Throw in all the nuts and seeds to the mixture and stir until well combined and nuts are fully coated.

4. Line a baking dish with parchment paper.

5. Pour mixture onto the baking dish and freeze for 20 minutes.

6. Remove the refrigerated nut base and spread the toppings and spread the extras over it.

7. Freeze for another hour then cut into bars and serve.

Keto Vegan Bagels

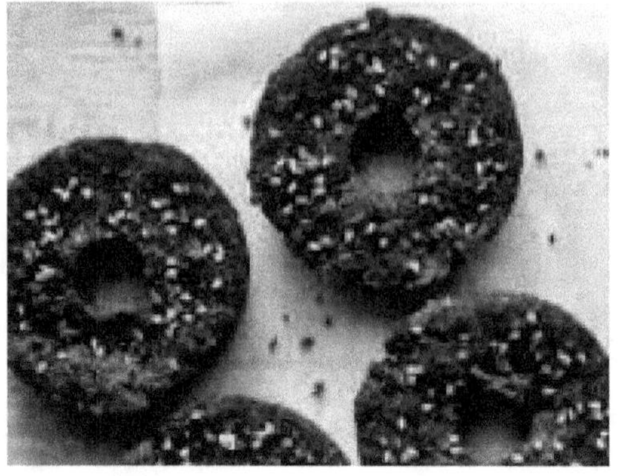

Preparation Time: 20 Minutes - Cooking Time: 40 Minutes - Servings: 6 – Calories : 308

Ingredients

- A pinch salt
- Half a cup of ground golden flaxseed
- Two (2) tablespoons of coconut oil (melted)
- One (1) teaspoon of baking powder
- A quarter cup of psyllium husk powder
- Half a cup of Almond butter (unsweetened and unsalted)

Toppings;

- A quarter teaspoon of salt
- One (1) teaspoon of sesame seeds
- One (1) teaspoon of dried onion flakes

- Six (6) tablespoons of vegan cream cheese
- One (1) teaspoon of dried garlic flakes
- One (1) teaspoon of poppy seeds

Directions:

For the bagels:

1. Preheat your oven to 375F
2. Use a tablespoon of coconut oil to grease the sections of a doughnut pan.
3. Put the baking powder, psyllium husk powder, salt and ground flax seed into a bowl, stir until well combined.
4. Put the almond butter into a large bowl, add a cup of warm water and whisk until smooth.
5. Add dry ingredients and stir until well combined until a moldable dough is formed.
6. Cut the dough into six portions and set aside.
7. For the toppings;
8. Put the sesame seeds, poppy seeds, sea salt, onion flakes and garlic flakes into a small bowl and stir to combine then set aside.

To bake :

9. Roll the dough into long logs by just rolling them back and forth, then press them into the greased molds.

10. Coat the top of bagels with the rest of the coconut oil using a marinating brush.

11. Sprinkle an even amount of the toppings over the bagels.

12. Bake for 40 minutes or until the bagels are a dark golden color.

13. Leave in the mold to cool in the tray before moving to a wire rack to cool completely.

14. Serve with some vegan cream cheese and enjoy.

Note: If the bagels do not cool well enough before being removed from the mold, they'll break, so let it cool in the mold for 10 minutes at least.

Keto Vegan Protein Bites

Preparation Time: 10 Minutes - Cooking Time: 10 Minutes - Servings: 16 – Calories : 249

Ingredients

For cookie dough base :

- Two (2) tablespoons of coconut oil
- A quarter cup of dairy free chocolate chips
- A quarter cup of Almond flour
- Half a cup of softened coconut butter or any nut seed butter of your choice
- Two (2) tablespoons of shredded coconut (unsweetened)
- Half a teaspoon of sea salt
- One (1) teaspoon of vanilla extract or two(2) teaspoons of vanilla bean powder
- Four (4) tablespoons of raw honey or maple syrup
- A quarter cup of vegan protein powder
- One (1) teaspoon of cinnamon
- For pumpkin spice flavor;
- Cookie dough base
- One (1) teaspoon of maple syrup
- Four (4) tablespoons of plain pumpkin puree(unsweetened)

- A quarter teaspoon of ground ginger
- Half a teaspoon of ground cinnamon
- One (1) tablespoon of Almond flour
- A pinch of ground mace
- Two (2) tablespoons of shredded coconut (unsweetened)
- Three (3) drops of liquid stevia
- A quarter teaspoon of ground cloves
- Chocolate mint flavor;
- Cookie dough base
- A quarter cup of shredded coconut (unsweetened)
- One (1) teaspoon of Peppermint extract
- Two (2) tablespoons of coconut oil
- Three (3) tablespoons of cocoa powder
- One (1) teaspoon of chopped pepper mint leaves
- One (1) teaspoon of maple syrup
- Chocolate cherry flavor;
- Cookie dough base
- One (1) teaspoon of maple syrup
- Two (2) tablespoons of coconut oil
- Two (2) tablespoons unsulfured dried cherries
- One (1) tablespoon of cocoa powder

Directions:

1. In a medium bowl, add but butter or coconut, honey or maple syrup, vanilla and coconut oil. Stir until fully combined.
2. Put in the dry ingredients and stir until well combined using the back of a spoon as the dough is very sticky. Put in the chocolate chips or any other flavoring.
3. Cut the dough into bite sized balls and role between the flat of your palms.
4. Line a baking dish or tray with pieces of parchment paper.
5. Transfer the rolled dough balls into a pre-lined baking sheet.
6. Refrigerate for an hour to get a firm chewy consistency.
7. Serve and enjoy.

Note: The bites can last for as long as a week if kept in an airtight container and refrigerated in a fixed temperature.

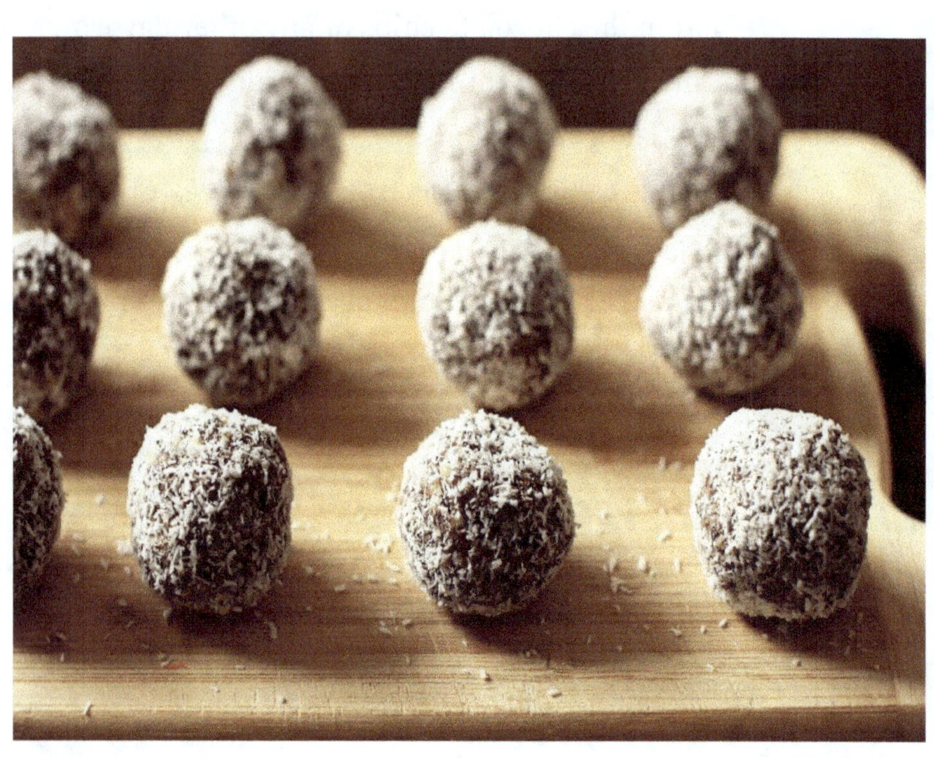

No-Bake Coconut Chia Macaroons

Preparation Time: 2 hours - Cooking Time: - Servings: 6

Ingredients:

- 1 cup Shredded Coconut
- 2 tbsp. Chia Seeds
- ½ cup Coconut Cream
- ½ cup Erythritol

Directions:

5. Combine all ingredients in a bowl. Mix until well combined.
6. Chill the mixture for about half an hour.
7. Once set, scoop the mixture into serving portions and roll into balls.
8. Return to the chiller for another hour.

Nutrition: Kcal per serve: 129 / Fat: 12 g. (80%) / Protein: 2 g. (5%) / Carbs: 5 g. (15%)

Avocado Lassi

A truly satisfying and refreshing smoothie that's sure to provide you with the nutrients your body needs. With recipes as simple as this, there's definitely no excuse to sticking to a healthy diet.

Preparation Time: 5 minutes - Cooking Time: - Servings: 3

Ingredients:

- 1 Avocado
- 1 cup Coconut Milk
- 2 cups Ice Cubes
- 2 tbsp. Erythritol
- ½ tsp Powdered Cardamom
- 1 tbsp. Vanilla Extract

Directions:

1. Combine all ingredients in a bowl. Mix until well combined.
2. Press the mixture into a rectangular silicon mold and freeze for an hour to set.
3. Slice for serving.

Nutrition: Kcal per serve: 305 / Fat: 29 g. (83%) / Protein: 3 g. (4%) / Carbs: 9 g. (13%)

Vegan Fudge Revel Bars

Preparation Time: 1 hour - Cooking Time: - Servings: 12

Ingredients:

- 1 cup Almond Flour
- ¾ cup Erythritol
- ¾ cup Peanut Butter
- 1 tbsp. Vanilla extract
- ½ cup Sugar-Free Chocolate Chips
- 2 tbsp. Margarine

Directions:

1. Mix together almond butter, coconut flour, erythritol, and vanilla extract in a bowl until well combined.
2. Press the mixture into a rectangular silicon mold and freeze for an hour to set.
3. Melt the chocolate chips with the margarine for 1-2 minutes in the microwave.
4. Pour melted chocolate on top of the mold and chill for another hour to set.
5. Slice for serving.

Nutrition: Kcal per serve: 160 / Fat: 14 g. (74%) / Protein: 5 g. (12%) / Carbs: 5 g. (14%)

Vegan Banana Bread

Preparation Time: 10 min - Cooking Time: 1 hour - Servings: 12

Ingredients:

- 2 cups Almond Flour - ¼ cup Coconut Flour
- 1 tbsp. Baking Powder - 1 tbsp. Cinnamon Powder
- ¼ tsp Salt - ¼cup Chopped Pecans
- ½ cup Coconut Oil - ½ cup Erythritol
- 4 Flax Eggs - ¼ cup Almond Milk
- 1 tbsp. Banana Extract

Directions:

1. Preheat oven to 350F.
2. Combine all ingredients in a blender and process until smooth.
3. Scrape the batter into a loaf pan lined with parchment. Top with chopped pecans.
4. Bake for 50-60 minutes.
5. Allow to cool before slicing.

Nutrition: Kcal per serve: 192 / Fat: 18 g. (82%) / Protein: 3 g. (7%) / Carbs: 6 g. (11%)

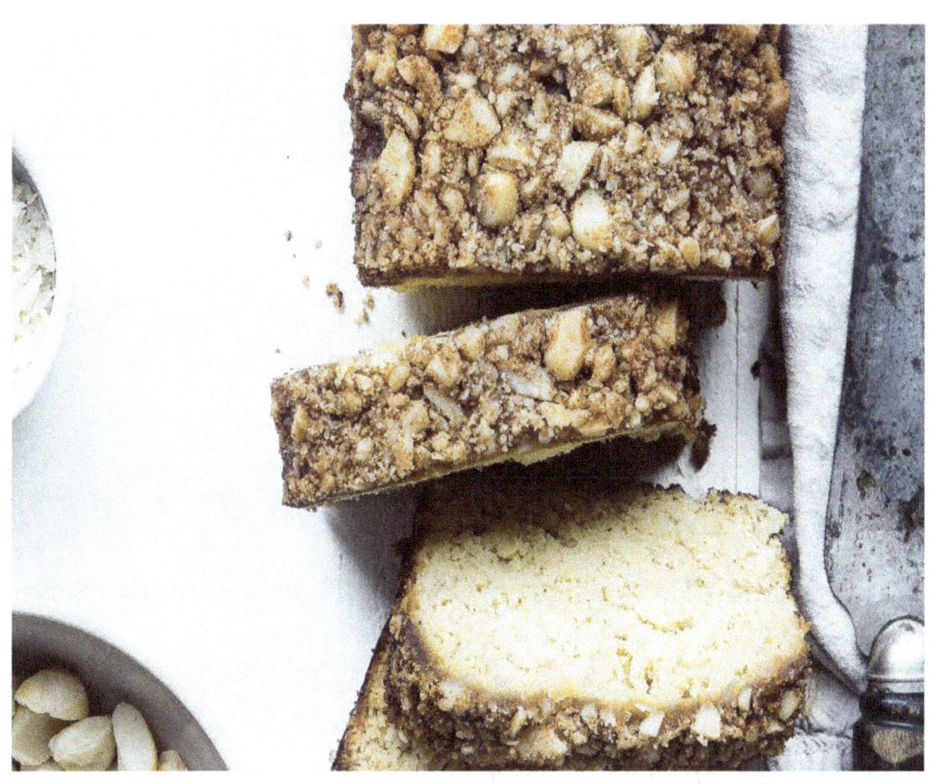

Bulgogi-Spiced Tofu Wraps

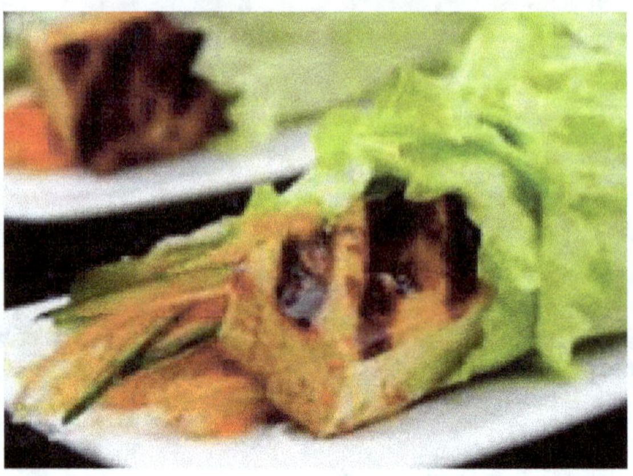

Preparation Time: 2 hours - Cooking Time: 5 minutes - Servings: 6

Ingredients:

- 400 g Firm Tofu
- 200 grams Iceberg Lettuce for wrapping

For the Marinade

- 50g chopped Leeks - 2 tbsp. Soy Sauce
- 1 tsp Erythritol - 2 tbsp. Sesame Oil

For the Slaw

- 50 g White Radish, julienne - 50 g Cucumber, julienne
- 50 g Carrots, julienne - 20 g Scallions, julienne

For the Dip:

- 1 tbsp. ml Light Soy sauce - 2 tbsp. ml Sesame oil
- 1 tsp Erythritol - 1 tbsp. Gochujang

Directions:

1. Combine all ingredients for the tofu marinade in a bowl. Whisk until fully combined.
2. Cut tofu into 1 inch thick slices and allow to marinate for not less than 2 hours.
3. While marinating prepare the slaw. Whisk all ingredients for the dressing. Toss in all chopped vegetables. Cover and refrigerate.
4. Grill the tofu and cut into approximately 1"x3" strips.
5. Toss chopped tofu with the prepared slaw.
6. Serve with lettuce leaves for wrapping.
7. Allow to cool before slicing.

Nutrition: Kcal per serve: 198 / Fat: 15 g. (66%) / Protein: 12 g. (21%) / Carbs: 7 g. (14%)

Vegan Baked Jelly Doughnuts

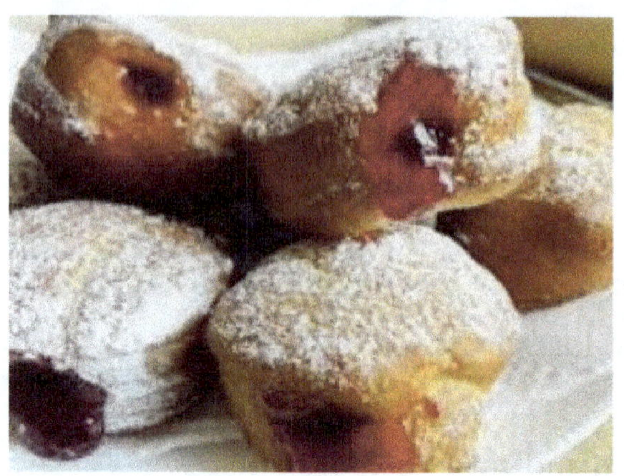

Preparation Time: 1.5 hours - Cooking Time: 10 minutes - S ervings: 12

Ingredients:

- 1 tbsp. Yeast - 2 tbsp. Warm Water
- 180 ml Soymilk - 1 tbsp. Erythritol Maple Syrup
- 1 gram Baking Soda - ¼tsp Salt
- 1 tbsp. Flaxseed Meal - 3 tbsp. Water
- 2 tbsp. Olive Oil - 500 grams Almond Flour
- 150 grams Desiccated Coconut - Sugar-Free Fruit Jelly(for filling)

Directions:

1. Sprinkle yeast over warm water and allow to bloom for about five minutes.
2. Stir flaxseed meal in water and bloom for 5 minutes.
3. In a large bowl, mix together yeast mixture, flaxseed mixture, soymilk, erythritol, and olive oil.
4. Whisk almond flour and baking soda in a separate bowl. Gradually beat flour into the wet ingredients.
5. Knead the resulting dough for about 5 minutes or until smooth and elastic.
6. Place the dough in a lightly oiled bowl and cover. Leave to rise for about an hour in a warm place.
7. Turn the dough onto a floured surface. Roll out into ½" thickness and cut into circles.
8. Transfer to a sheet pan, cover, and leave again to rise for another hour.
9. Bake for 8-10 minutes at 420F.
10. Place on a rack to cool.
11. Fill each doughnut with your choice of jelly using a pastry injector.
12. Coat with desiccated coconut.

Nutrition: Kcal per serve: 251 / Fat: 22 g. (71%) / Protein: 9 g. (14%) / Carbs: 9 g. (15%)

Curry-Spiked Vegetable Latkes

Preparation Time: 15 minutes - Cooking Time: 6 minutes - Servings: 6

Ingredients:

- 100 grams Carrots, spiralized - 100 grams Zucchini, spiralized
- 100 grams Cauliflower, minced - 50 grams White Onion, minced
- 5 grams Parsley, chopped - ¼ cup Almond Flour
- 1 tbsp. Flax Seeds, soaked in 2 tbsp. Water - 2 tsp Curry Powder
- ½ tsp Salt - 2 tbsp. Olive Oil plus more for frying

Directions:

1. Mix shredded vegetables, onions, parsley, almond flour, egg, salt, and curry powder in a bowl.
2. Heat olive oil in a non-stick skillet.
3. Spoon the vegetable mixture into the hot oil, shaping each latke with an egg ring.
4. Fry the latkes for 3 minutes per side over medium heat.
5. Drain on paper towels.

Nutrition: Kcal per serve: 123 / Fat: 12 g. (80%) / Protein: 2 g. (5%) / Carbs: 5 g. (15%)

Keto Cheese Bread

Preparation Time: 9 minutes - Cooking Time: 25 minutes - Servings: 6

Ingredients:

- 1 teaspoon Baking Powder - ¼ teaspoon Salt
- 1/3 cup Milk - 1 cup Almond Flour
- 2 large Whole Eggs - ½ cup Grated Parmesan
- 1/3 cup Cream Cheese, softened

Directions:

1. Preheat oven to 350°F.
2. Whisk together almond flour, baking powder, and salt in a bowl.
3. In a separate, bowl beat eggs and add cream cheese. Gradually stir in the milk.
4. Stir the wet mixture into the dry ingredients.
5. Fold in the grated parmesan.
6. Coat a 6-hole muffin tin with non-stick spray.
7. Divide the batter into the pan and bake for 25 minutes.

Nutrition: Calories 203 / Carbohydrates 6 g / Fats 16 g / Protein 9 g

Keto Hummus Quesadillas

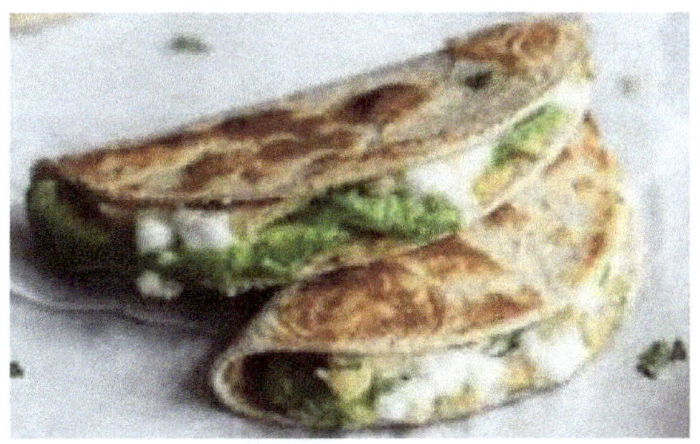

Have been craving for a hot quesadilla for quite some time but can't find a vegan alternative? This keto snack may just be the recipe you've been looking for.

Preparation Time: 20 min - Cooking Time: 20 minutes - Servings: 6

Ingredients:

For the Hummus

- 200 grams Cauliflower
- ¼ cup Olive Oil
- 1 tbsp. Lemon Juice
- 1 tbsp. Curry Powder
- 1 clove Garlic, minced
- ½ tsp Salt
- ¼ tsp Chili Powder

For the Flatbread:

- ½ cup Almond Flour

- 2 tbsp. Psyllium Husk

- ¼ tsp Baking Soda

- pinch of Salt

- 1 tbsp. Olive Oil

- 1 cup Lukewarm Water

Directions:

Prepare the Flatbread:

1. Whisk together the almond flour, psyllium husk, baking soda, and salt in a bowl.
2. Add in the water and olive oil.
3. Knead until everything comes together into a smooth dough.
4. Leave to rest for about 15 minutes.
5. Divide the dough into 6 equal-sized portions.
6. Roll each portion into a ball, then flatten with a rolling pin in between sheets of parchment paper.
7. Refrigerate until ready to use.
8. To cook, heat in a non-stick pan for 2-3 minutes per side.

Prepare the hummus:

9. Boil cauliflower for 5 minutes, or until tender. Drain.

10. Put cauliflower in a food processor together with the rest of the ingredients for the hummus in a food processor. Blend until smooth.

Assemble the tortillas:

11. Take a piece of flatbread.
12. Spread a generous amount of prepared hummus to one side.
13. Fold the tortilla in half.
14. Toast the filled tortillas for 1-2 minutes each side in a non-stick skillet.
15. Slice up and serve.

Nutrition: Kcal per serve: 158 / Fat: 15 g. (85%) / Protein: 2 g. (5%) / Carbs: 4 g. (10%)

Keto Mug Bread

Preparation Time: 2 minutes - Cooking Time: 2 minutes - Servings: 1

Ingredients:

- 1/3 cup Almond Flour
- ½ tsp Baking Powder
- ¼ tsp Salt
- 1 Whole Egg
- 1 tbsp. Melted Butter

Directions:

1. Mix all ingredients in a microwave-safe mug.
2. Microwave for 90 seconds.
3. Cool for 2 minutes.

Nutrition: Calories 416 / Carbohydrates 8 g / Fats 37 g / Protein 15 g

Avocado Stuffed with Tomato and Mushrooms

Preparation Time: 10 minutes - Cooking Time: 10 minutes - Servings: 4

Ingredients

- 4 avocados, pitted and halved
- 2 tablespoons olive oil
- 2 cups button mushrooms, chopped
- 1 onion, chopped
- 1 teaspoon garlic, crushed
- Salt and black pepper, to taste
- 1 teaspoon deli mustard
- 1 tomato, chopped

Directions

1. Scoop out about 2 teaspoons of avocado flesh from each half; reserve the scooped avocado flash.
2. Heat the oil in a sauté pan that is preheated over a moderately high flame. Now, cook the mushrooms, onion, and garlic until the mushrooms are tender and the onion is translucent.

3. Add the reserved avocado flash to the mushroom mixture and mix to combine. Now, add the salt, black pepper, mustard, and tomato.
4. Divide the mushroom mixture among the avocado halves and serve immediately.

Nutrition: 245 Calories / 23.2g Fat / 8.2g Carbs / 2.4g Protein / 7.5g Fiber

Tofu-Kale Dip with Crudités

Preparation Time: 15 minutes - Cooking Time: 25 minutes - Servings: 2

Ingredients

- 2 cups kale
- 1 cup tofu, pressed, drained and crumbled
- 1/2 cup soy milk
- 2 teaspoons nutritional yeast
- 2 garlic cloves, minced
- 2 teaspoons olive oil
- 1 teaspoon sea salt
- 1/4 teaspoon ground black pepper, or more to taste
- 1/2 teaspoon paprika
- 1 teaspoon dried basil
- 1/2 teaspoon dried dill weed

Directions

1. Start by preheating your oven to 400 degrees F. Lightly oil a casserole dish with a nonstick cooking spray.
2. Now, parboil the kale leaves until it is just wilted.

3. Puree the remaining ingredients in your food processor or blender. Stir in the kale; stir until the mixture is homogeneous.

4. Bake approximately 13 minutes. Now, serve with a crudités platter. Bon appétit!

Nutrition: 75 Calories / 3g Fat / 5g Carbs / 2.9g Protein / 1.2g Fiber

Keto Blender Buns

Preparation Time: 5 minutes - Cooking Time: 25 minutes - Servings: 6

Ingredients:

- 4 Whole Eggs
- ¼ cup Melted Butter
- ½ tsp Salt
- ½ cup Almond Flour
- 1 tsp Italian Spice Mix

Directions:

1. Preheat oven to 425°F.
2. Pulse all ingredients in a blender.
3. Divide batter into a 6-hole muffin tin.
4. Bake for 25 minutes.

Nutrition: Calories 200 / Carbohydrates 2 g / Fats 18 g / Protein 8 g

Keto Burger Buns

Preparation Time: 10 minutes - Cooking Time: 12 minutes - Servings: 6

Ingredients:

- 1 cup Almond Flour
- ¼ cup Psyllium Husk Powder
- 1 tsp Baking Powder
- 1 cup Mozzarella Cheese
- ¼ cup Cream Cheese
- 1 Egg - tbsp. Sesame Seeds

Directions:

1. Preheat oven to 400°F.
2. Melt the two cheeses together in the microwave.
3. Blend the melted cheese together then stir in the egg.
4. Whisk together the almond flour, psyllium husk, and baking powder in a separate bowl.
5. Mix the dry ingredients into the cheese mixture until a dough is formed.
6. Divide the dough into 6 and roll each portion into a ball.
7. Top each ball with sesame seeds.

8. Arrange on a baking sheet lined with parchment and bake for 12 minutes.

9. Leave to cool for 10-15 minutes before slicing into halves.

Nutrition: Calories 216 / Carbohydrates 5 g / Fats 18 g / Protein 10 g

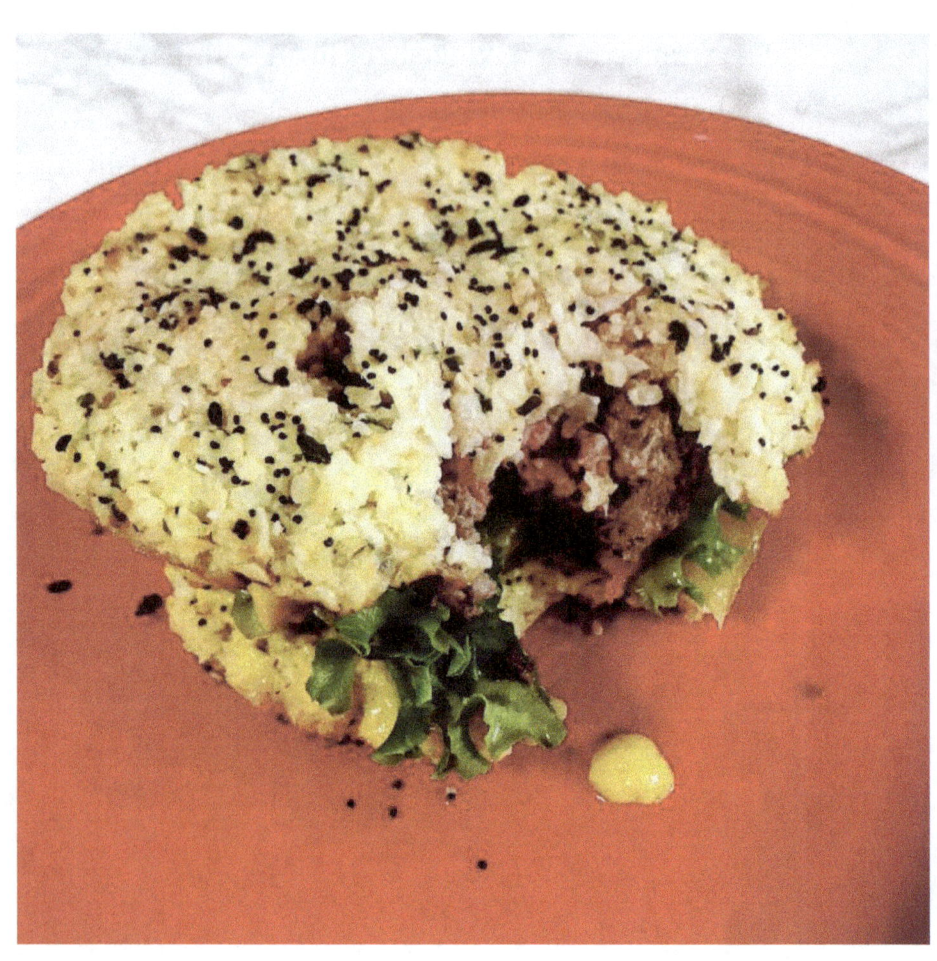

Keto Pizza Crust

Preparation Time: 10 minutes - Cooking Time: 6 minutes - Servings: 8

Ingredients:

- 1 cup Almond Flour
- 2 cups Shredded Mozzarella
- 2 tbsp. Cream Cheese
- pinch of Salt

Directions:

1. Combine both cheeses in a bowl and melt in the microwave.
2. Stir then gradually knead in the salt and almond flour.
3. Roll out to flatten in between sheets of parchment.
4. Bake at 350°F for 6 minutes.
5. Put choice of toppings on and bake for another 5-10 minutes.

Nutrition: Calories 165 / Carbohydrates 3 g / Fats 13 g / Protein 9 g

Coco-Cilantro Flatbread

Preparation Time: 10 minutes - Cooking Time: 15 minutes - Servings: 6

Ingredients:

- ½ cup Coconut Flour
- 2 tablespoons Flax Meal
- ¼ teaspoon Baking Soda
- 1 tablespoon Coconut Oil
- 2 tablespoons Chopped Cilantro
- ¼ teaspoon salt
- 1 cup Lukewarm Water

Directions:

1. In a medium bowl, whisk together the coconut flour, flax, baking soda, and salt.
2. Add in the water, coconut oil, and chopped cilantro.
3. Knead until everything comes together into a smooth dough.
4. Leave to rest for about 15 minutes.
5. Divide the dough into 6 equal-sized portions.
6. Roll each portion into a ball, then flatten with a rolling pin in between sheets of parchment paper.

7. Refrigerate until ready to use.

8. To cook, heat in a non-stick pan for 2-3 minutes per side.

Nutrition: Calories 46 / Carbohydrates 1 g / Fats 4 g / Protein 1 g

Avocado Flatbread

Preparation Time: 25 minutes - Cooking Time: 5 minutes - Servings: 6

Ingredients:

- 130 grams Mashed Avocado
- ¾ cup Chickpea Flour
- 1 tsp Cumin Powder
- ½ tsp Salt

Directions:

1. Combine all ingredients in a bowl. Stir until mixture comes together into a dough.
2. Knead the dough briefly on a lightly floured surface.
3. Leave the dough to rest for 15 minutes.
4. Divide the dough into four portions.
5. Take each portion of dough and flatten with a rolling pin.
6. Toast flatbread in a lightly oiled skillet for about 2 minutes per side.

Nutrition: Calories 80 / Carbohydrates 8 g / Fats 4 g / Protein 3 g

Keto hamburger buns

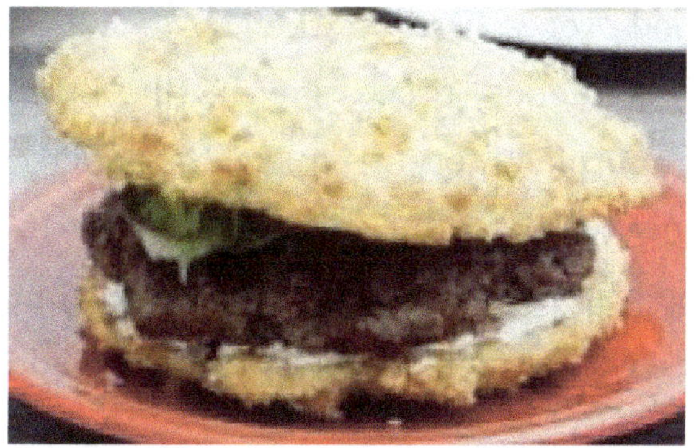

Preparation Time: 5 minutes - Cooking Time: 15 minutes - Servings: 5

Ingredients:

- 1 1/4 cup almond flour
- 1 1/2 cup mozzarella cheese, part skim grated
- 2 oz. cream cheese
- 1 egg, large
- 2 tablespoons oat fiber 500/ protein powder
- 1 tablespoon baking powder
- 1 Metal plate or a pan which you care less about

Directions:

1. Using a microwave safe bowl, put the cream cheese and mozzarella cheese. Microwave the cheese for I minutes. Remove the bowl, stir and microwave again for 40 seconds to another minute.

2. Scrape out the cheese and place it together with the egg into a food processor. Stop when it's smooth. Add your dry ingredients, processing it till dough is formed. (It is normally very sticky) Let the dough cool.

3. Preheat your oven to 400°F, placing the rack in the middle. Line your baking sheet with parchment paper and place the cheap metal plate or pan at the bottom of the oven.

4. Once the oven is ready, separate the dough into 5 equal portions. Apply oil on your hands (not too much) and roll the portions into balls. Place them on the parchment paper, flattening them a bit while creating a domed shape.

5. Put 5 or 6 ice cubes on the metal pan and place the buns inside the oven. The steam from the cubes will make the buns rise.

6. Bake them for about fifteen minutes. They should be done once they brown on the outside. If not, give them more minutes in the oven.

Nutrition: Calories 294 / Carbohydrates 7 g / Fats 25 g / Protein 14 g

Paleo, Keto buns

Preparation Time: 10 minutes - Cooking Time: 45 minutes - Servings: 10

Ingredients:

- 1 1/2 cup almond meal - 1/2 cup coconut flour
- 1/2 cup flax meal - 2/3 cup psyllium husks
- 6 egg whites, large - 2 eggs, large
- 5 tablespoons sesame seeds
- 2 teaspoons garlic powder
- 2 teaspoons cream of tartar/ apple cider vinegar
- 2 teaspoon onion powder
- 1 teaspoon baking soda
- 1 teaspoon sea salt/ pink Himalayan
- 2 tablespoons Erythritol
- 480 ml boiling water

Directions:

1. Preheat your oven to 350°F
2. Mix all your dry ingredients in a mixing bowl.
3. Add your egg whites and eggs. Use a hand mixer to process it till your dough becomes thick.
4. Add the boiling water and process until it combines.
5. Line your baking sheet with parchment paper.

6. Use a spoon to make the buns and create a dome shape.

7. Sprinkle the sesame seeds on the buns. Press the seeds into the buns to prevent them from falling out.

8. Bake for 45 minutes.

Nutrition: Calories 208 / Carbohydrates 9 g / Fats 12 g / Protein 6 g

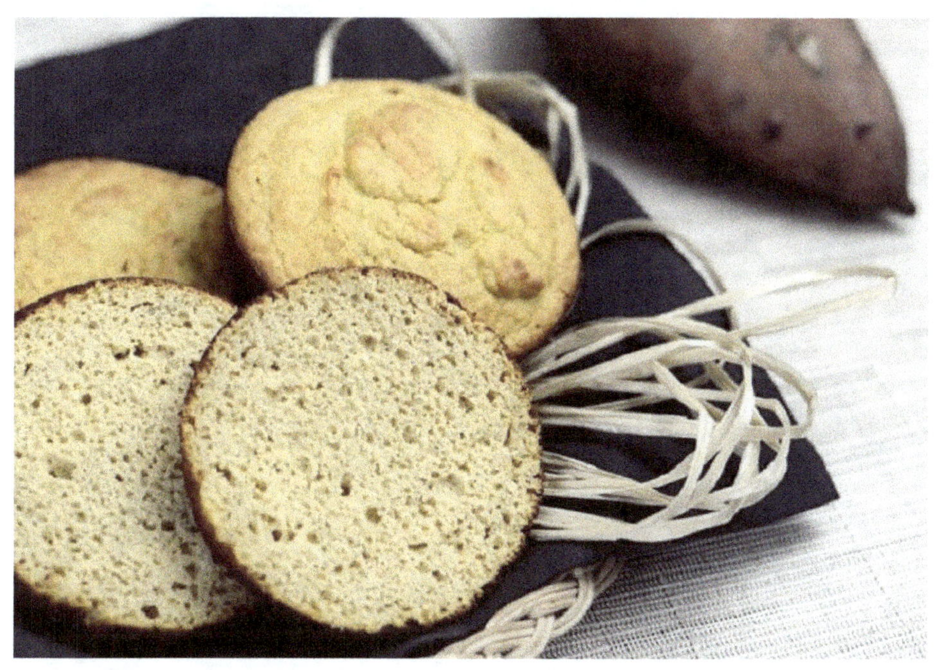